ANESTHESIA ESSENTIALS

Real Scenarios, Real Solutions

Essam Abdelhakim

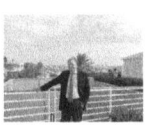

Copyright © 2024 Essam Abdelhakim

All rights reserved

The characters and events portrayed in this book are fictitious. Any similarity to real persons, living or dead, is coincidental and not intended by the author.

No part of this book may be reproduced, or stored in a retrieval system, or transmitted in any form or by any means, electronic, mechanical, photocopying, recording, or otherwise, without express written permission of the publisher.

Cover design by: Art Painter
Library of Congress Control Number: 2018675309
Printed in the United States of America

CONTENTS

Title Page
Copyright
Introduction
Disclosure

1. Scenario: Difficult Airway	1
2. Scenario: Malignant Hyperthermia	2
3. Scenario: Spinal Anesthesia in a Parturient	3
4. Scenario: Anaphylaxis During Induction	4
5. Scenario: Local Anesthetic Toxicity	5
6. Scenario: Hypoxia in One-Lung Ventilation	6
7. Scenario: Emergence Delirium	7
8. Scenario: Postoperative Nausea and Vomiting (PONV)	8
9. Scenario: Aspiration During Induction	9
10. Scenario: Bradycardia During Spinal Anesthesia	10
11. Scenario: Hypotension after Induction	11
12. Scenario: Failed Epidural Analgesia	12
13. Scenario: Obstructive Sleep Apnea (OSA) in Anesthesia	13
14. Scenario: Delayed Emergence	14
15. Scenario: Accidental Dural Puncture During Epidural	15
16. Scenario: Anesthesia for a Patient with Myasthenia Gravis	16

17. Scenario: Bradycardia during Laparoscopic Surgery	17
18. Scenario: Acute Pain in a Chronic Opioid User	18
19. Scenario: Tachycardia and Hypertension During Surgery	19
20. Scenario: Hypoxia in a Pediatric Patient	20
21. Scenario: Awake Craniotomy	21
22. Scenario: Hypothermia in the OR	22
23. Scenario: Patient with Cardiac Stents	23
24. Scenario: Hyperkalemia and Succinylcholine	24
25. Scenario: Intraoperative Awareness	25
26. Scenario: Transfusion Reaction	26
27. Scenario: Local Anesthetic Failure in a Peripheral Nerve Block	27
28. Scenario: Anesthesia for Obese Patients	28
29. Scenario: Compartment Syndrome after Surgery	29
30. Scenario: Prolonged Paralysis after Neuromuscular Blockade	30
31. Scenario: Difficult Airway and Can't Intubate, Can't Ventilate (CICV)	31
32. Scenario: Pheochromocytoma Crisis during Surgery	32
33. Scenario: Hyperkalemia after Succinylcholine in a Burn Patient	33
34. Scenario: Perioperative Myocardial Infarction	34
35. Scenario: Local Anesthetic Systemic Toxicity (LAST)	35
36. Scenario: Postoperative Vision Loss	36
37. Scenario: Thyroid Storm during Surgery	37
38. Scenario: Postoperative Delirium	38
39. Scenario: Post-Dural Puncture Headache (PDPH)	39
40. Scenario: Difficult Extubation after Thyroidectomy	40
41. Scenario: Negative Pressure Pulmonary Edema (NPPE)	41

42. Scenario: Failed Spinal Anesthesia in Obese Patient — 42
43. Scenario: Aortic Dissection in the OR — 43
44. Scenario: Intraoperative Air Embolism — 44
45. Scenario: Perioperative Stroke — 45
46. Scenario: Laryngospasm in a Pediatric Patient — 46
47. Scenario: Congenital Diaphragmatic Hernia (CDH) in a Neonate — 47
48. Scenario: Inhalational Induction in a Pediatric Patient — 48
49. Scenario: Airway Obstruction in a Child with a Respiratory Infection — 49
50. Scenario: Foreign Body Aspiration in a Child — 50
51. Scenario: Sickle Cell Crisis in a Pediatric Patient — 51
52. Scenario: Pediatric Anesthesia for a Patient with Trisomy 21 — 52
53. Scenario: Caudal Epidural for Pediatric Pain Management — 53
54. Scenario: Pediatric Blood Loss in Surgery — 54
55. Scenario: Hypotension after Spinal Anesthesia for Cesarean Section — 55
56. Scenario: Difficult Airway in a Pregnant Patient — 56
57. Scenario: Uterine Atony and Hemorrhage after Delivery — 57
58. Scenario: Amniotic Fluid Embolism (AFE) — 58
59. Scenario: Airway Management in a Patient with Large Thyroid Mass — 59
60. Scenario: Superior Vena Cava Syndrome (SVCS) — 60
61. Scenario: Anesthetic Management for Intracranial Tumor Resection — 61
62. Scenario: Paraneoplastic Syndrome in Anesthesia — 62
63. Scenario: Chemotherapy-Induced Cardiotoxicity — 63
64. Scenario: Anesthetic Management for a Patient with Leukemia — 64

65. Scenario: Radiation-Induced Fibrosis in Airway Management — 65

66. Scenario: Hypercalcemia in a Patient with Multiple Myeloma — 66

67. Scenario: Perioperative Management in a Patient with Lung Cancer and Chronic Obstructive Pulmona — 67

68. Scenario: Intraoperative Tumor Lysis Syndrome — 68

69. Scenario: Hypotension in a Trauma Patient with Pelvic Fracture — 69

70. Scenario: Airway Management in a Patient with Cervical Spine Injury — 70

71. Scenario: Hemorrhagic Shock from Liver Laceration — 71

72. Scenario: Massive Transfusion Protocol in Trauma — 72

73. Scenario: Tension Pneumothorax during Trauma Surgery — 73

74. Scenario: Acute Respiratory Distress Syndrome (ARDS) — 74

75. Scenario: Weaning from Mechanical Ventilation — 75

76. Scenario: Ventilator-Associated Pneumonia (VAP) — 76

77. Scenario: Patient with Chronic Obstructive Pulmonary Disease (COPD) on Ventilator — 77

78. Scenario: Patient with Acute Asthma Exacerbation on Mechanical Ventilation — 78

79. Scenario: Ventilator Management in Obese Patients — 79

80. Scenario: Patient with Sepsis on Mechanical Ventilation — 80

81. Scenario: Non-Invasive Ventilation (NIV) for Acute Pulmonary Edema — 81

82. Scenario: Ventilator Management in a Patient with Traumatic Brain Injury (TBI) — 82

83. Scenario: Acute Hypercapnic Respiratory Failure in Neuromuscular Disease — 83

84. Scenario: Acute Postoperative Pain Management	84
85. Scenario: Chronic Pain Management with Neuropathic Component	85
86. Scenario: Cancer Pain Management	86
87. Scenario: Labor Analgesia	87
88. Scenario: Acute Pain Management in a Trauma Patient	88
89. Scenario: Pain Management for a Patient with Complex Regional Pain Syndrome (CRPS)	89
90. Scenario: Chronic Low Back Pain Management	90
91. Scenario: Pain Control in Patients with Sickle Cell Crisis	91
92. Scenario: Regional Anesthesia for Ambulatory Surgery	92
93. Scenario: Pediatric Pain Management During Surgery	93
94. Scenario: Pain Management in Preterm Infant During Procedures	94
95. Scenario: Managing Pain in a Neonate with NEC	95
96. Scenario: Pain Management in Neonatal Intubation	96
97. Scenario: Postoperative Pain Management in Neonates	97
98. Scenario: Pain Management for Neonates with Withdrawal Symptoms	98
99. Scenario: Managing Pain from Phototherapy in Jaundiced Neonates	99
100. Scenario: Pain Assessment in a Critically Ill Neonate	100
101. Scenario: Pain Management During Central Line Insertion	101
102. Scenario: Managing Pain for a Neonate with Cardiac Issues	102
103. Scenario: Long-term Pain Management in a NICU Patient	103
104. Scenario: Anesthesia for Coronary Artery Bypass Grafting (CABG)	104

105. Scenario: Intraoperative Hypotension During Surgery — 105

106. Scenario: Awareness Under General Anesthesia — 106

107. Scenario: Management of Anticoagulation in Cardiac Surgery — 107

108. Scenario: Cardiopulmonary Bypass Complications — 108

109. Scenario: Acute Coronary Syndrome (ACS) During Surgery — 109

110. Scenario: Hemolytic Reaction During Cardiac Surgery — 110

111. Scenario: Intraoperative Cardiac Arrest — 111

112. Scenario: Anesthesia for Craniotomy — 112

113. Scenario: Intraoperative Neuromonitoring — 113

114. Scenario: Postoperative Cerebral Edema — 114

115. Scenario: Seizure Management in Neurosurgery — 115

116. Scenario: Anesthesia for Spinal Fusion — 116

117. Scenario: Anesthesia for Thyroidectomy — 117

118. Scenario: Hyperparathyroidism Surgery Complications — 118

119. Scenario: Postoperative Hypoparathyroidism — 119

120. Scenario: Cardiovascular Instability During Endocrine Surgery — 120

121. Scenario: Anesthesia for Patient with Chronic Kidney Disease (CKD) — 121

122. Scenario: Intraoperative Hemolysis in a Dialysis Patient — 122

123. Scenario: Postoperative Management of a Patient with Acute Kidney Injury (AKI) — 123

124. Scenario: Anesthesia for Renal Transplantation — 124

125. Scenario: Managing Electrolyte Imbalance in a Dialysis Patient — 125

126. Scenario: Anesthesia for Liver Transplantation — 126

127. Scenario: Postoperative Complications Following Kidney Transplant — 127

128. Scenario: Intraoperative Anaphylaxis During Heart Transplant — 128

129. Scenario: Management of Hyperglycemia in a Pancreas Transplant — 129

130. Scenario: Postoperative Care for Lung Transplant Patient — 130

About The Author — 131

INTRODUCTION

Clinical Scenarios in Anesthesia: A Comprehensive Guide for Medical Doctors and Residents

This book is designed as an essential resource for medical doctors and residents specializing in anesthesia. It presents a collection of clinical scenarios that encapsulate the complexities and challenges faced in various surgical settings. Covering a wide range of topics, including neurosurgery, endocrine surgery, renal disorders, and transplant procedures, each scenario is meticulously crafted to enhance the reader's clinical reasoning and decision-making skills.

The book provides detailed descriptions of patient cases, highlighting key anesthetic considerations, potential complications, and management strategies. Each scenario is accompanied by answers, explanations, and practical tips, offering insights into best practices and fostering a deeper understanding of the anesthetic management of diverse patient populations.

With a focus on real-world applications, this guide aims to prepare readers for the dynamic and often unpredictable nature of the operating room. It serves not only as a valuable educational tool for residents but also as a quick reference for practicing anesthesiologists. By bridging the gap between theoretical knowledge and practical experience, this book equips its readers with the necessary skills to ensure patient safety and optimize surgical outcomes.

Whether preparing for exams, enhancing clinical skills, or navigating daily practice, *Clinical Scenarios in Anesthesia* is an indispensable companion for those dedicated to the field of anesthesiology.

DISCLOSURE

Disclosure

This book has been created with the assistance of *Artificial Intelligence (AI) tools* and thoroughly reviewed and edited by the author to ensure clarity, relevance, and educational value.

While every effort has been made to provide accurate and up-to-date information, this content is intended solely for educational and informational purposes.

The author is a medical professional; however, the information provided in this book *is not a substitute for professional medical advice, diagnosis, or treatment.*

Readers are strongly advised to consult licensed healthcare providers or specialists for any medical concerns or conditions.

By using this book, **you acknowledge and agree** that the author shall not be held responsible or liable for any loss, damage, or harm whether physical, emotional, financial, or otherwise that may occur *as a result of the use or misuse of the information presented herein.*

1. SCENARIO: DIFFICULT AIRWAY

A 45-year-old male with a BMI of 40 requires emergency surgery for a perforated peptic ulcer. During the pre-anesthesia assessment, you suspect a difficult airway due to his short neck, large tongue, and limited mouth opening. How do you manage the airway?

- **Answer**: Perform awake fiberoptic intubation or use a video laryngoscope.
- **Explanation**: Obesity and anatomical variations suggest a difficult airway. Awake fiberoptic intubation allows continuous airway assessment, and video laryngoscopes can improve visualization.
- **Tip**: Always prepare for surgical airway backup (e.g., cricothyrotomy) in suspected difficult airway cases.

2. SCENARIO: MALIGNANT HYPERTHERMIA

A 28-year-old male is undergoing general anesthesia for elective shoulder surgery. Shortly after the administration of sevoflurane, his heart rate increases to 140 bpm, and his end-tidal CO_2 rises. His temperature spikes to 40°C. What is the diagnosis, and how should it be managed?

- **Answer**: Malignant hyperthermia; administer dantrolene and discontinue triggering agents.
- **Explanation**: Malignant hyperthermia is a life-threatening hypermetabolic state triggered by volatile anesthetics or succinylcholine. Dantrolene is the specific antidote.
- **Tip**: Early recognition and rapid administration of dantrolene are key to survival.

3. SCENARIO: SPINAL ANESTHESIA IN A PARTURIENT

A 32-year-old pregnant woman at 38 weeks gestation presents for an elective cesarean section. Spinal anesthesia is chosen. Shortly after injection, she develops hypotension and bradycardia. What is the most likely cause and treatment?

- **Answer**: Sympathetic blockade causing hypotension; treat with vasopressors (e.g., ephedrine or phenylephrine).
- **Explanation**: Spinal anesthesia causes sympathetic blockade, leading to vasodilation, hypotension, and bradycardia. Vasopressors restore vascular tone and improve hemodynamics.
- **Tip**: Preload with IV fluids and monitor blood pressure closely after spinal anesthesia.

4. SCENARIO: ANAPHYLAXIS DURING INDUCTION

During induction of general anesthesia, a 40-year-old female suddenly develops hypotension, bronchospasm, and a rash after receiving rocuronium. What is the likely diagnosis, and what are the immediate steps in management?

- **Answer**: Anaphylaxis; administer epinephrine, fluids, and antihistamines.
- **Explanation**: Anaphylaxis is a severe allergic reaction that can occur during anesthesia, especially to muscle relaxants like rocuronium. Epinephrine reverses bronchospasm and hypotension.
- **Tip**: Always have an anaphylaxis kit ready with epinephrine, corticosteroids, and antihistamines.

5. SCENARIO: LOCAL ANESTHETIC TOXICITY

A 60-year-old male receives a peripheral nerve block with bupivacaine for knee surgery. Shortly after, he becomes confused, seizes, and has cardiac arrest. What is the diagnosis, and how is it treated?

- **Answer**: Local anesthetic systemic toxicity (LAST); treat with IV lipid emulsion therapy.
- **Explanation**: Bupivacaine is cardiotoxic in high concentrations, leading to seizures and cardiac arrest. Lipid emulsion therapy acts as a "lipid sink" to bind the local anesthetic.
- **Tip**: Always calculate the maximum safe dose of local anesthetics and monitor closely after administration.

6. SCENARIO: HYPOXIA IN ONE-LUNG VENTILATION

A 55-year-old male is undergoing thoracotomy for lung cancer resection. During one-lung ventilation, his oxygen saturation drops to 85%. What is the first step in managing hypoxia in this patient?

- **Answer**: Increase the fraction of inspired oxygen (FiO2) and apply positive end-expiratory pressure (PEEP) to the ventilated lung.
- **Explanation**: Hypoxia during one-lung ventilation occurs due to ventilation-perfusion mismatch. Increasing FiO2 and applying PEEP can improve oxygenation.
- **Tip**: If hypoxia persists, consider reinflating the non-ventilated lung or using CPAP.

7. SCENARIO: EMERGENCE DELIRIUM

A 4-year-old boy is recovering from general anesthesia for tonsillectomy. He becomes agitated, crying, and thrashing around. What is the likely diagnosis, and how should it be managed?

- **Answer**: Emergence delirium; manage with reassurance and, if necessary, small doses of midazolam or dexmedetomidine.
- **Explanation**: Emergence delirium is common in pediatric patients, especially after sevoflurane anesthesia. It typically resolves spontaneously but can be distressing for the patient and family.
- **Tip**: Preventive measures include using propofol or dexmedetomidine during the anesthetic.

8. SCENARIO: POSTOPERATIVE NAUSEA AND VOMITING (PONV)

A 30-year-old female with a history of motion sickness and nonsmoking status undergoes laparoscopic cholecystectomy. She experiences severe nausea and vomiting in the recovery room. How do you prevent and treat PONV?

- **Answer**: Administer ondansetron and dexamethasone prophylactically, treat with additional antiemetics (e.g., metoclopramide) postoperatively.
- **Explanation**: Risk factors for PONV include female gender, history of motion sickness, nonsmoking status, and volatile anesthetics. Ondansetron (5-HT3 antagonist) and dexamethasone are effective in prevention.
- **Tip**: Use a multimodal approach to PONV prevention in high-risk patients.

9. SCENARIO: ASPIRATION DURING INDUCTION

A 70-year-old male with a history of GERD is undergoing emergency surgery. During rapid sequence induction, he vomits and aspirates. What is your immediate management?

- **Answer**: Suction the airway, administer oxygen, and consider intubation with a cuffed tube to protect the lungs.
- **Explanation**: Aspiration during anesthesia is a life-threatening complication that can lead to aspiration pneumonitis. Immediate airway management and suctioning are critical.
- **Tip**: Preoxygenation and rapid sequence induction (RSI) with cricoid pressure reduce the risk of aspiration.

10. SCENARIO: BRADYCARDIA DURING SPINAL ANESTHESIA

A 65-year-old male undergoing transurethral resection of the prostate under spinal anesthesia suddenly develops bradycardia (HR 40 bpm). What is the cause, and how do you manage it?

- **Answer**: Sympathetic blockade affecting cardiac accelerator fibers; treat with atropine.
- **Explanation**: Spinal anesthesia can block sympathetic fibers, leading to unopposed parasympathetic stimulation and bradycardia. Atropine is an anticholinergic that increases heart rate.
- **Tip**: Monitor heart rate closely after spinal anesthesia, especially in older patients.

11. SCENARIO: HYPOTENSION AFTER INDUCTION

A 60-year-old female with a history of hypertension and diabetes undergoes induction of general anesthesia for a hip replacement. Shortly after propofol and fentanyl administration, her blood pressure drops to 75/45 mmHg. How do you manage this hypotension?

- **Answer**: Administer IV fluids and vasopressors (e.g., phenylephrine or ephedrine).
- **Explanation**: Propofol causes vasodilation and reduces systemic vascular resistance, leading to hypotension. IV fluids and vasopressors restore hemodynamic stability.
- **Tip**: Consider using lower doses of induction agents in elderly or high-risk patients to minimize hypotension.

12. SCENARIO: FAILED EPIDURAL ANALGESIA

A 35-year-old woman is in active labor and requests epidural analgesia. After placement, she continues to feel intense pain on one side of her abdomen. What could be the cause, and how would you manage it?

- **Answer**: Unilateral block due to catheter malposition; adjust the catheter or administer a bolus of local anesthetic.
- **Explanation**: Unilateral pain is often due to improper catheter placement or inadequate spread of the local anesthetic. Adjusting the catheter or giving an additional dose can resolve the issue.
- **Tip**: Test the epidural block level using ice or pinprick to ensure adequate pain control on both sides.

13. SCENARIO: OBSTRUCTIVE SLEEP APNEA (OSA) IN ANESTHESIA

A 50-year-old male with a history of severe obstructive sleep apnea (OSA) is scheduled for elective hernia repair under general anesthesia. How would you modify your anesthesia plan for this patient?

- **Answer**: Use regional anesthesia if possible, avoid opioids, and closely monitor postoperatively for respiratory depression.
- **Explanation**: OSA patients are at increased risk for airway obstruction and postoperative respiratory complications. Minimizing opioid use and opting for regional techniques can reduce these risks.
- **Tip**: Postoperative continuous positive airway pressure (CPAP) should be continued for patients with OSA.

14. SCENARIO: DELAYED EMERGENCE

A 70-year-old male undergoes general anesthesia for abdominal surgery. After surgery, he remains unresponsive for over 45 minutes in the recovery room. What is your differential diagnosis, and how would you manage it?

- **Answer**: Differential includes residual anesthetic effects, hypothermia, electrolyte imbalance, or stroke; assess with blood gases, electrolytes, and neurology review.
- **Explanation**: Delayed emergence can be caused by lingering effects of anesthetics, especially in older patients, or by metabolic disturbances. Immediate evaluation is necessary to rule out life-threatening causes.
- **Tip**: Reassess all medications administered and ensure normothermia before extubation.

15. SCENARIO: ACCIDENTAL DURAL PUNCTURE DURING EPIDURAL

A 32-year-old woman receives an epidural for labor pain. The anesthetist accidentally punctures the dura, and the patient reports a severe headache after delivery. What is the cause, and how would you treat it?

- **Answer**: Post-dural puncture headache (PDPH); treat with conservative measures (hydration, caffeine) or an epidural blood patch if severe.
- **Explanation**: PDPH occurs due to CSF leakage from the punctured dura, leading to decreased intracranial pressure. An epidural blood patch seals the hole and alleviates symptoms.
- **Tip**: Inform patients about the risk of PDPH after a dural puncture and ensure they are aware of treatment options.

16. SCENARIO: ANESTHESIA FOR A PATIENT WITH MYASTHENIA GRAVIS

A 55-year-old female with myasthenia gravis is scheduled for thymectomy under general anesthesia. How should her anesthetic management be modified?

- **Answer**: Minimize or avoid neuromuscular blocking agents, and carefully titrate non-depolarizing agents if needed.

- **Explanation**: Myasthenia gravis patients have increased sensitivity to muscle relaxants, which can lead to prolonged paralysis. Use of short-acting anesthetics and minimal relaxant doses is preferred.

- **Tip**: Consider using a nerve stimulator to monitor neuromuscular function intraoperatively.

17. SCENARIO: BRADYCARDIA DURING LAPAROSCOPIC SURGERY

A 40-year-old male undergoes laparoscopic cholecystectomy under general anesthesia. During insufflation of the abdomen with CO2, his heart rate drops to 40 bpm. What is the most likely cause, and how would you manage it?

- **Answer**: Vagal stimulation due to peritoneal stretching; reduce insufflation pressure and administer atropine if necessary.
- **Explanation**: Peritoneal insufflation during laparoscopy can stimulate the vagus nerve, causing bradycardia. Reducing the pressure and giving anticholinergics can counteract this effect.
- **Tip**: Monitor heart rate closely during insufflation, and keep atropine available for treatment.

18. SCENARIO: ACUTE PAIN IN A CHRONIC OPIOID USER

A 45-year-old male with chronic back pain on high-dose opioids presents for elective spine surgery. Postoperatively, he complains of severe pain despite standard doses of analgesics. How would you manage his postoperative pain?

- **Answer**: Administer higher doses of opioids or consider using multimodal analgesia with regional techniques.
- **Explanation**: Chronic opioid users often develop tolerance, requiring higher doses for pain relief. Regional anesthesia or adjuvant medications like ketamine can improve analgesia.
- **Tip**: Preoperatively discuss the plan for managing opioid-tolerant patients with the surgical and pain management teams.

19. SCENARIO: TACHYCARDIA AND HYPERTENSION DURING SURGERY

A 65-year-old male with a history of coronary artery disease and hypertension is undergoing abdominal surgery. During the procedure, he develops tachycardia (HR 120 bpm) and hypertension (BP 180/100 mmHg). What are the possible causes, and how would you manage it?

- **Answer**: Possible causes include inadequate anesthesia, pain, or fluid overload; deepen anesthesia, treat with opioids or beta-blockers.
- **Explanation**: Intraoperative tachycardia and hypertension can be due to inadequate depth of anesthesia or surgical stimulation. Adjusting anesthetic depth and treating with short-acting agents like esmolol may help.
- **Tip**: Always assess anesthetic depth and monitor vital signs frequently during surgery.

20. SCENARIO: HYPOXIA IN A PEDIATRIC PATIENT

A 2-year-old child is undergoing tonsillectomy under general anesthesia. During the procedure, the oxygen saturation drops to 88%. What are the possible causes, and how would you manage it?

- **Answer**: Possible causes include airway obstruction, bronchospasm, or hypoventilation; check the airway and provide supplemental oxygen or bronchodilators if necessary.

- **Explanation**: Pediatric patients are prone to airway obstruction and hypoxia during anesthesia due to their smaller airways. Quick assessment and intervention are crucial to prevent further desaturation.

- **Tip**: Use a pediatric-sized airway device and monitor ventilation closely in younger patients.

21. SCENARIO: AWAKE CRANIOTOMY

A 35-year-old male is scheduled for an awake craniotomy for tumor resection in the motor cortex. What anesthetic approach would you use to ensure patient comfort while maintaining neurological monitoring?

- **Answer**: Use local anesthesia with sedation (dexmedetomidine or propofol) and allow for intermittent awakening during neurological testing.
- **Explanation**: Awake craniotomy requires the patient to be responsive for motor function testing while the surgeon operates. Sedation should be titrated to maintain cooperation and airway protection.
- **Tip**: Plan for meticulous airway management and have a strategy for quick conversion to general anesthesia if needed.

22. SCENARIO: HYPOTHERMIA IN THE OR

A 70-year-old female undergoes a 6-hour abdominal surgery. By the end of the procedure, her body temperature is 34°C. What complications could arise, and how would you manage it?

- **Answer**: Hypothermia can cause coagulopathy, delayed drug metabolism, and cardiac arrhythmias; use active warming measures such as forced-air warming blankets and warmed IV fluids.
- **Explanation**: Hypothermia during surgery is associated with increased bleeding, delayed recovery, and wound infections. Active warming is essential to avoid complications.
- **Tip**: Monitor temperature throughout long surgeries and start active warming early.

23. SCENARIO: PATIENT WITH CARDIAC STENTS

A 65-year-old male with coronary artery stents placed 6 months ago requires non-cardiac surgery. He is on aspirin and clopidogrel. How should you manage his antiplatelet therapy before surgery?

- **Answer**: Continue aspirin and discontinue clopidogrel 5-7 days before surgery; if surgery is urgent, consider bridging with short-acting antiplatelets or heparin.
- **Explanation**: Discontinuing both antiplatelets increases the risk of stent thrombosis, but dual antiplatelet therapy increases the risk of bleeding during surgery. Aspirin is usually continued to maintain some antiplatelet effect.
- **Tip**: Collaborate with cardiology to plan the safest strategy for patients with recent stents.

24. SCENARIO: HYPERKALEMIA AND SUCCINYLCHOLINE

A 40-year-old male with chronic renal failure presents for emergency surgery. His preoperative potassium is 6.2 mmol/L. Should you use succinylcholine for rapid sequence intubation?

- **Answer**: No, avoid succinylcholine and use a non-depolarizing muscle relaxant like rocuronium.
- **Explanation**: Succinylcholine can cause a transient rise in serum potassium, which may exacerbate hyperkalemia and lead to life-threatening arrhythmias. Non-depolarizing agents are safer in patients with elevated potassium.
- **Tip**: Always check electrolyte levels before using succinylcholine, especially in patients with renal failure or crush injuries.

25. SCENARIO: INTRAOPERATIVE AWARENESS

A 50-year-old woman undergoing laparoscopic hysterectomy under general anesthesia reports being aware during surgery and hearing voices. What are the risk factors, and how would you prevent this in future cases?

- **Answer**: Risk factors include low-dose anesthetics, inadequate monitoring, and patient factors like opioid tolerance; prevent by ensuring adequate depth of anesthesia and using monitoring like bispectral index (BIS).
- **Explanation**: Intraoperative awareness occurs when the depth of anesthesia is insufficient to suppress consciousness. Ensuring proper anesthetic dosing and using BIS monitoring reduces this risk.
- **Tip**: Discuss awareness with patients during preoperative counseling, especially if they have risk factors.

26. SCENARIO: TRANSFUSION REACTION

A 60-year-old male undergoes hip replacement and receives a blood transfusion intraoperatively. He develops fever, hypotension, and dark urine. What is the likely diagnosis, and how should you manage it?

- **Answer**: Acute hemolytic transfusion reaction; stop the transfusion immediately, administer IV fluids, and support blood pressure with vasopressors if necessary.
- **Explanation**: Hemolytic reactions occur when incompatible blood is transfused, leading to red cell destruction. Immediate cessation of the transfusion and supportive care are critical.
- **Tip**: Always double-check patient identification and blood type before administering a transfusion.

27. SCENARIO: LOCAL ANESTHETIC FAILURE IN A PERIPHERAL NERVE BLOCK

A 45-year-old male is scheduled for shoulder surgery under an interscalene block. Despite proper technique, the patient reports full sensation in the arm 30 minutes after the block. What might have gone wrong, and how would you proceed?

- **Answer**: Possible failure of the block due to incomplete spread of the local anesthetic or wrong needle placement; repeat the block or convert to general anesthesia.

- **Explanation**: Incomplete nerve blockade can occur due to anatomical variations or inadequate drug spread. Repeating the block or switching to general anesthesia ensures adequate pain control.

- **Tip**: Use ultrasound guidance to confirm needle position and local anesthetic spread during peripheral nerve blocks.

28. SCENARIO: ANESTHESIA FOR OBESE PATIENTS

A 45-year-old female with a BMI of 45 presents for laparoscopic cholecystectomy. What are the anesthetic considerations for obese patients?

- **Answer**: Plan for difficult airway management, avoid high doses of opioids, and consider postoperative ventilation support.
- **Explanation**: Obesity increases the risk of difficult airway, respiratory depression, and postoperative hypoxia. Regional anesthesia and non-opioid analgesics can reduce respiratory complications.
- **Tip**: Position obese patients with head elevation during induction to improve oxygenation and airway management.

29. SCENARIO: COMPARTMENT SYNDROME AFTER SURGERY

A 30-year-old male undergoes open reduction and internal fixation of a tibial fracture. In the recovery room, he complains of severe pain in his leg that is out of proportion to the injury. What is your diagnosis, and how do you proceed?

- **Answer**: Suspected compartment syndrome; consult orthopedics for immediate fasciotomy.
- **Explanation**: Compartment syndrome is a surgical emergency where increased pressure within a muscle compartment compromises blood flow and nerve function. Urgent fasciotomy is required to prevent permanent damage.
- **Tip**: Monitor postoperative pain closely, especially after orthopedic surgeries, as disproportionate pain is a key sign of compartment syndrome.

30. SCENARIO: PROLONGED PARALYSIS AFTER NEUROMUSCULAR BLOCKADE

A 55-year-old male undergoing general anesthesia for abdominal surgery receives rocuronium for muscle relaxation. Postoperatively, he fails to regain muscle strength and remains paralyzed. What is the cause, and how should you treat it?

- **Answer**: Suspected prolonged neuromuscular blockade due to inadequate reversal or pseudocholinesterase deficiency; administer sugammadex if rocuronium was used, or neostigmine for other agents.
- **Explanation**: Prolonged paralysis can result from residual neuromuscular blockade or enzymatic deficiencies. Sugammadex rapidly reverses rocuronium-induced paralysis, while neostigmine is used for other agents.
- **Tip**: Use neuromuscular monitoring (train-of-four) to ensure adequate recovery from paralysis before extubation.

31. SCENARIO: DIFFICULT AIRWAY AND CAN'T INTUBATE, CAN'T VENTILATE (CICV)

A 55-year-old male with a history of neck radiation presents for an emergency laparotomy. After induction, you are unable to intubate despite several attempts, and mask ventilation is ineffective. How would you manage this airway emergency?

- **Answer**: Initiate emergency front-of-neck access (cricothyroidotomy) and oxygenate the patient.
- **Explanation**: CICV is a critical airway emergency where neither intubation nor ventilation is possible. Cricothyroidotomy is the definitive lifesaving measure to secure the airway and restore oxygenation.
- **Tip**: Always have an emergency airway plan, and be prepared to perform a cricothyroidotomy in difficult airway scenarios.

32. SCENARIO: PHEOCHROMOCYTOMA CRISIS DURING SURGERY

A 50-year-old female with undiagnosed pheochromocytoma undergoes surgery. During tumor manipulation, her blood pressure skyrockets to 240/140 mmHg, and she becomes tachycardic. What is the diagnosis, and how would you manage this crisis?

- **Answer**: Hypertensive crisis due to pheochromocytoma; administer an alpha-blocker (e.g., phentolamine) and avoid beta-blockers until alpha blockade is established.

- **Explanation**: Pheochromocytomas release catecholamines, causing severe hypertension during surgery. Alpha-blockers reduce the vasoconstriction and prevent unopposed alpha stimulation if beta-blockers are used.

- **Tip**: Preoperative screening for pheochromocytoma is essential for patients with refractory hypertension or suggestive symptoms.

33. SCENARIO: HYPERKALEMIA AFTER SUCCINYLCHOLINE IN A BURN PATIENT

A 30-year-old male with 50% body surface area burns from 5 days ago is undergoing surgery for debridement. Succinylcholine is used for rapid sequence intubation, and within minutes the patient develops peaked T waves and bradycardia. What is the likely diagnosis, and how would you manage it?

- **Answer**: Hyperkalemia induced by succinylcholine; treat with IV calcium gluconate, insulin with glucose, and consider dialysis if refractory.
- **Explanation**: Burn patients are at risk for hyperkalemia after succinylcholine due to upregulation of extrajunctional acetylcholine receptors, causing massive potassium release. Non-depolarizing muscle relaxants are preferred in these patients.
- **Tip**: Avoid succinylcholine in patients with burns, crush injuries, or neuromuscular disorders, as they are prone to life-threatening hyperkalemia.

34. SCENARIO: PERIOPERATIVE MYOCARDIAL INFARCTION

A 70-year-old male with a history of coronary artery disease undergoes hip replacement. During surgery, he develops ST-segment depression on the ECG, hypotension, and chest pain. How would you manage this perioperative myocardial infarction?

- **Answer**: Administer nitroglycerin, optimize hemodynamics with fluids and inotropes, and consult cardiology for further management, including possible angiography.

- **Explanation**: Perioperative myocardial infarction (MI) can occur due to the stress of surgery, leading to ischemia. Immediate treatment with nitrates and hemodynamic optimization is crucial to limit damage.

- **Tip**: Patients with known coronary artery disease may benefit from preoperative risk stratification and perioperative beta-blockers.

35. SCENARIO: LOCAL ANESTHETIC SYSTEMIC TOXICITY (LAST)

A 45-year-old woman receives an interscalene block with bupivacaine for shoulder surgery. Shortly after injection, she becomes confused, seizes, and develops bradycardia. What is the diagnosis, and how would you treat it?

- **Answer**: Local anesthetic systemic toxicity (LAST); immediately stop the anesthetic, administer intravenous lipid emulsion, manage seizures with benzodiazepines, and provide cardiovascular support.
- **Explanation**: LAST occurs when high doses of local anesthetics enter the systemic circulation, causing CNS and cardiovascular toxicity. Lipid emulsion acts as a "lipid sink" to absorb the anesthetic and reverse toxicity.
- **Tip**: Use ultrasound guidance during nerve blocks to minimize the risk of intravascular injection, and have lipid emulsion readily available.

36. SCENARIO: POSTOPERATIVE VISION LOSS

A 65-year-old male undergoes prolonged spine surgery in the prone position. Postoperatively, he reports complete loss of vision in one eye. What is the diagnosis, and what factors contribute to this condition?

- **Answer**: Ischemic optic neuropathy (ION); contributing factors include prolonged prone positioning, hypotension, blood loss, and anemia.
- **Explanation**: ION is a rare but devastating complication of surgeries, particularly in the prone position, leading to reduced blood flow to the optic nerve. Risk reduction strategies include maintaining normal blood pressure and minimizing blood loss.
- **Tip**: Use careful positioning and intraoperative hemodynamic management to reduce the risk of ION in high-risk surgeries.

37. SCENARIO: THYROID STORM DURING SURGERY

A 45-year-old female with undiagnosed hyperthyroidism undergoes surgery. During the procedure, she develops severe tachycardia (HR 160), hyperthermia, and agitation. What is the diagnosis, and how would you manage it?

- **Answer**: Thyroid storm; treat with beta-blockers (e.g., propranolol), antithyroid medications (e.g., propylthiouracil), and corticosteroids. Cool the patient and provide supportive care.
- **Explanation**: Thyroid storm is a life-threatening exacerbation of hyperthyroidism, triggered by surgery or stress. Beta-blockers control tachycardia, while antithyroid drugs reduce thyroid hormone synthesis.
- **Tip**: Screen for hyperthyroidism in patients with signs of thyrotoxicosis, especially if undergoing stressful procedures.

38. SCENARIO: POSTOPERATIVE DELIRIUM

An 80-year-old male with a history of dementia undergoes hip fracture repair. Postoperatively, he becomes agitated, confused, and disoriented. What is the likely diagnosis, and how would you manage this patient?

- **Answer**: Postoperative delirium; manage with a calm environment, minimize sedatives, and treat any underlying causes such as infection or electrolyte imbalances.
- **Explanation**: Postoperative delirium is common in elderly patients, particularly those with preexisting cognitive impairment. Non-pharmacological strategies like reorientation and sleep promotion are effective.
- **Tip**: Avoid excessive sedation in elderly patients and encourage early mobilization to reduce the incidence of delirium.

39. SCENARIO: POST-DURAL PUNCTURE HEADACHE (PDPH)

A 35-year-old woman undergoes a cesarean section under spinal anesthesia. On postoperative day 2, she complains of severe headache that worsens when sitting or standing and improves when lying flat. What is your diagnosis, and how would you manage it?

- **Answer**: Post-dural puncture headache (PDPH); manage with conservative measures like hydration, caffeine, and analgesics, or perform an epidural blood patch if symptoms persist.
- **Explanation**: PDPH occurs due to cerebrospinal fluid (CSF) leakage through the dural puncture site, causing traction on intracranial structures when upright. An epidural blood patch seals the puncture and alleviates symptoms.
- **Tip**: Use small-gauge, pencil-point spinal needles to reduce the risk of PDPH.

40. SCENARIO: DIFFICULT EXTUBATION AFTER THYROIDECTOMY

A 50-year-old female undergoes a total thyroidectomy for thyroid cancer. Postoperatively, you plan for extubation but notice significant neck swelling. How would you manage this situation?

- **Answer**: Suspect a neck hematoma; immediately reintubate and prepare for surgical evacuation of the hematoma.
- **Explanation**: Post-thyroidectomy neck hematoma can compromise the airway, leading to life-threatening airway obstruction. Early recognition and prompt intervention are critical.
- **Tip**: In high-risk cases, delay extubation until airway swelling is ruled out or resolved.

41. SCENARIO: NEGATIVE PRESSURE PULMONARY EDEMA (NPPE)

A 30-year-old healthy male undergoes elective shoulder surgery under general anesthesia. Postoperatively, after extubation, he develops sudden respiratory distress with frothy pink sputum. What is your diagnosis, and how would you manage it?

- **Answer**: Negative pressure pulmonary edema (NPPE); manage with supplemental oxygen, non-invasive ventilation, and diuretics if necessary.
- **Explanation**: NPPE is caused by upper airway obstruction (e.g., laryngospasm) after extubation, creating negative intrathoracic pressure that leads to fluid leakage into the alveoli.
- **Tip**: Be cautious during extubation, especially in younger, healthy patients, as they generate high negative pressure during obstruction, increasing the risk for NPPE.

42. SCENARIO: FAILED SPINAL ANESTHESIA IN OBESE PATIENT

A 40-year-old obese female (BMI 45) is scheduled for a cesarean section under spinal anesthesia. Despite two attempts at spinal anesthesia, the block is inadequate. How would you proceed?

- **Answer**: Convert to general anesthesia or attempt a combined spinal-epidural (CSE) technique if feasible.
- **Explanation**: Obesity makes spinal anesthesia technically difficult due to poor anatomical landmarks and increased epidural space. A CSE allows more flexibility in dosing and provides an option to convert to epidural if the spinal fails.
- **Tip**: Consider early use of ultrasound to locate landmarks in obese patients, and have a plan for failed regional anesthesia.

43. SCENARIO: AORTIC DISSECTION IN THE OR

A 65-year-old male with hypertension develops sudden severe chest and back pain during induction for a routine surgery. Blood pressure becomes difficult to control. What is your diagnosis, and how would you manage this?

- **Answer**: Suspect aortic dissection; immediately suspend surgery, control blood pressure with beta-blockers and vasodilators, and consult vascular surgery for emergency intervention.
- **Explanation**: Aortic dissection is a life-threatening condition that requires rapid diagnosis and blood pressure control to prevent rupture. Definitive treatment involves surgical repair.
- **Tip**: In patients with risk factors for aortic dissection (e.g., hypertension, connective tissue disease), be vigilant for signs of chest or back pain during anesthesia.

44. SCENARIO: INTRAOPERATIVE AIR EMBOLISM

A 55-year-old female undergoes neurosurgery in the sitting position. Suddenly, her end-tidal CO_2 drops, and she becomes hypotensive. What is your diagnosis, and how would you manage it?

- **Answer**: Suspect venous air embolism; immediately lower the head of the bed, flood the surgical field with saline, aspirate air from the central venous catheter (if present), and provide 100% oxygen.

- **Explanation**: Venous air embolism occurs when air enters the circulation, typically during surgery in the sitting position. Prompt intervention is required to prevent cardiovascular collapse.

- **Tip**: Continuously monitor for air embolism with end-tidal CO_2 and precordial Doppler in high-risk cases like neurosurgery in the sitting position.

45. SCENARIO: PERIOPERATIVE STROKE

A 75-year-old male with a history of atrial fibrillation and hypertension undergoes carotid endarterectomy. Postoperatively, he is unable to move his right arm and has slurred speech. What is the likely diagnosis, and how would you manage it?

- **Answer**: Suspect perioperative stroke; immediately consult neurology for evaluation and consider thrombolytic therapy if within the appropriate time window.
- **Explanation**: Perioperative strokes are more common in vascular surgeries and in patients with cardiovascular risk factors. Rapid assessment and intervention can reduce long-term deficits.
- **Tip**: Preoperative optimization of stroke risk factors (e.g., anticoagulation for atrial fibrillation) and early postoperative neurological monitoring are crucial for stroke prevention.

46. SCENARIO: LARYNGOSPASM IN A PEDIATRIC PATIENT

A 4-year-old boy is undergoing tonsillectomy under general anesthesia. Shortly after extubation, the patient develops stridor and desaturation. What is your diagnosis, and how would you manage it?

- **Answer**: Laryngospasm; treat with positive pressure ventilation and, if unresolved, administer IV succinylcholine (0.1-0.2 mg/kg) or deepen anesthesia.
- **Explanation**: Laryngospasm is a common complication in pediatric patients, particularly after airway surgeries. It involves the involuntary closure of the vocal cords, leading to airway obstruction.
- **Tip**: Prevent laryngospasm by ensuring the patient is in a deep plane of anesthesia during airway manipulation and by using suction to clear secretions.

47. SCENARIO: CONGENITAL DIAPHRAGMATIC HERNIA (CDH) IN A NEONATE

A newborn with a prenatal diagnosis of CDH is scheduled for immediate surgical repair. During anesthesia, the neonate develops severe hypoxemia and decreased lung compliance. How would you manage this?

- **Answer**: Avoid overventilation of the hypoplastic lung, use low tidal volumes, high-frequency oscillatory ventilation if needed, and maintain gentle ventilation strategies.
- **Explanation**: CDH involves abdominal organs herniating into the thorax, impairing lung development. Aggressive ventilation can cause barotrauma and worsen the condition.
- **Tip**: In neonates with CDH, carefully balance ventilation to avoid overinflating the affected lung, and maintain adequate oxygenation through gentle respiratory support.

48. SCENARIO: INHALATIONAL INDUCTION IN A PEDIATRIC PATIENT

A 2-year-old child with no IV access is undergoing an urgent procedure. How would you safely induce anesthesia in this patient?

- **Answer**: Perform inhalational induction using sevoflurane with gradual increases in concentration.
- **Explanation**: Inhalational induction is the preferred method for children, as it avoids the distress associated with IV placement. Sevoflurane is well-tolerated and has a rapid onset.
- **Tip**: Use distraction techniques like blowing bubbles or watching cartoons to help the child remain calm during induction.

49. SCENARIO: AIRWAY OBSTRUCTION IN A CHILD WITH A RESPIRATORY INFECTION

A 3-year-old boy with a recent upper respiratory tract infection (URI) is scheduled for adenotonsillectomy. After extubation, he develops severe respiratory distress. What is your diagnosis, and how would you manage this?

- **Answer**: Post-extubation croup; treat with nebulized epinephrine and IV dexamethasone.
- **Explanation**: Children with recent URIs are at higher risk for airway edema and post-extubation croup, particularly after airway surgeries.
- **Tip**: Delay elective surgery in children with recent URIs to reduce the risk of airway complications, and use corticosteroids prophylactically when surgery cannot be postponed.

50. SCENARIO: FOREIGN BODY ASPIRATION IN A CHILD

A 5-year-old boy presents with sudden onset of coughing, wheezing, and decreased breath sounds on the right side during a dental procedure under general anesthesia. What would be your diagnosis, and how would you manage it?

- **Answer**: Suspect foreign body aspiration; immediately secure the airway, prepare for rigid bronchoscopy, and maintain spontaneous ventilation until the foreign body is retrieved.
- **Explanation**: Foreign body aspiration in children can cause life-threatening airway obstruction, requiring prompt diagnosis and intervention, often with bronchoscopy.
- **Tip**: Avoid positive pressure ventilation until the airway is secured, as it may push the foreign body deeper into the lungs.

51. SCENARIO: SICKLE CELL CRISIS IN A PEDIATRIC PATIENT

A 10-year-old girl with sickle cell disease is scheduled for an appendectomy. During induction, she complains of severe pain in her legs and arms. What is your diagnosis, and how would you manage it?

- **Answer**: Sickle cell crisis; administer oxygen, hydrate the patient, provide analgesia, and consider transfusion if necessary.
- **Explanation**: Sickle cell crises can be triggered by stress, dehydration, and hypoxia during anesthesia. Maintaining adequate hydration and oxygenation is essential to prevent complications.
- **Tip**: Avoid hypothermia and acidosis, and use a multidisciplinary approach, including hematology input, to manage sickle cell patients perioperatively.

52. SCENARIO: PEDIATRIC ANESTHESIA FOR A PATIENT WITH TRISOMY 21

A 5-year-old child with trisomy 21 (Down syndrome) is scheduled for a cardiac procedure. What special considerations should you keep in mind during anesthesia?

- **Answer**: Consider a difficult airway due to macroglossia and subglottic stenosis, as well as the risk of bradycardia during airway manipulation.
- **Explanation**: Children with trisomy 21 often have challenging airways and cardiac abnormalities. Bradycardia can occur during intubation due to increased vagal tone.
- **Tip**: Use smaller endotracheal tubes, have airway adjuncts ready, and monitor closely for cardiac complications.

53. SCENARIO: CAUDAL EPIDURAL FOR PEDIATRIC PAIN MANAGEMENT

A 6-year-old boy is undergoing circumcision. You plan to use a caudal block for postoperative analgesia. What are the key considerations in performing a caudal block in pediatric patients?

- **Answer**: Use appropriate dosing based on weight (e.g., 0.5-1 mL/kg of local anesthetic), and ensure the block is performed under sterile conditions to avoid infection.
- **Explanation**: The caudal block provides excellent postoperative analgesia for lower abdominal and urogenital surgeries in children, reducing the need for systemic opioids.
- **Tip**: Always aspirate before injecting to avoid intravascular injection, and monitor for signs of local anesthetic toxicity.

54. SCENARIO: PEDIATRIC BLOOD LOSS IN SURGERY

A 3-year-old child is undergoing a major abdominal procedure. Intraoperatively, you notice significant blood loss. What is the best way to estimate the allowable blood loss and manage it?

- **Answer**: Calculate allowable blood loss using the child's estimated blood volume (EBV: 80 mL/kg for children), monitor hematocrit, and replace blood with crystalloids, colloids, or blood products as needed.
- **Explanation**: Children have lower circulating blood volumes, and even small amounts of blood loss can lead to significant hemodynamic instability.
- **Tip**: Monitor blood loss closely in pediatric patients, and be ready to transfuse early if signs of hypovolemia or anemia develop.

55. SCENARIO: HYPOTENSION AFTER SPINAL ANESTHESIA FOR CESAREAN SECTION

A 30-year-old healthy pregnant woman receives spinal anesthesia for an elective cesarean section. Shortly after the spinal block, she develops significant hypotension. How would you manage it?

- **Answer**: Administer intravenous fluids, vasopressors (e.g., phenylephrine or ephedrine), and ensure left uterine displacement to improve venous return.
- **Explanation**: Hypotension after spinal anesthesia is common in obstetric patients due to vasodilation and decreased venous return. Prompt treatment is essential to maintain uteroplacental perfusion.
- **Tip**: Prophylactic vasopressors and fluid loading can reduce the incidence of hypotension after spinal anesthesia.

56. SCENARIO: DIFFICULT AIRWAY IN A PREGNANT PATIENT

A 35-year-old woman presents for an emergency cesarean section under general anesthesia. During induction, you encounter a difficult airway. How would you manage it?

- **Answer**: Use rapid sequence induction with cricoid pressure, avoid multiple intubation attempts, and be prepared to use a supraglottic airway or perform a surgical airway if needed.
- **Explanation**: Pregnant women are at increased risk for difficult airways due to airway edema and decreased functional residual capacity.
- **Tip**: Always have difficult airway equipment ready when managing obstetric patients, and consider early use of awake fiberoptic intubation in known difficult airways.

57. SCENARIO: UTERINE ATONY AND HEMORRHAGE AFTER DELIVERY

A 28-year-old woman undergoes a cesarean section for breech presentation. After the delivery of the baby, the uterus fails to contract, and she begins to bleed heavily. How would you manage this?

- **Answer**: Administer uterotonics (e.g., oxytocin, methylergonovine, or carboprost), initiate fluid resuscitation, and consider surgical interventions (e.g., uterine artery ligation or hysterectomy) if bleeding persists.
- **Explanation**: Uterine atony is the most common cause of postpartum hemorrhage, and timely administration of uterotonics is critical for controlling bleeding.
- **Tip**: Always have a postpartum hemorrhage protocol in place and be prepared for rapid transfusion if needed.

58. SCENARIO: AMNIOTIC FLUID EMBOLISM (AFE)

A 32-year-old woman in labor suddenly develops respiratory distress, hypotension, and cardiac arrest. What is your diagnosis, and how would you manage it?

- **Answer**: Suspect amniotic fluid embolism; initiate immediate cardiopulmonary resuscitation (CPR), provide oxygen, and consider transfusion of blood products to manage disseminated intravascular coagulation (DIC).

- **Explanation**: AFE is a rare but life-threatening obstetric emergency caused by the entry of amniotic fluid into the maternal circulation, leading to cardiovascular collapse and coagulopathy.

- **Tip**: Early recognition and aggressive supportive care are key to survival in AFE. Multidisciplinary management is essential.

59. SCENARIO: AIRWAY MANAGEMENT IN A PATIENT WITH LARGE THYROID MASS

A 55-year-old female patient with a large thyroid mass compressing the trachea presents for a thyroidectomy. You plan for general anesthesia. How would you approach airway management?

- **Answer**: Perform awake fiberoptic intubation with local anesthesia, avoiding muscle relaxants until the airway is secured.
- **Explanation**: Large thyroid masses may compress the trachea, increasing the risk of difficult intubation. Awake fiberoptic intubation maintains spontaneous ventilation and ensures control of the airway.
- **Tip**: Preoperative imaging to assess tracheal compression and having a surgical team ready for emergency tracheostomy are essential steps.

60. SCENARIO: SUPERIOR VENA CAVA SYNDROME (SVCS)

A 60-year-old male with a history of lung cancer and superior vena cava syndrome presents for a mediastinal mass biopsy. He complains of facial swelling and dyspnea. What are the anesthesia concerns and management?

- **Answer**: Avoid supine positioning, use gentle induction to prevent cardiovascular collapse, and consider local anesthesia if feasible.
- **Explanation**: SVCS reduces venous return, and the supine position may exacerbate airway and cardiovascular compromise.
- **Tip**: Keep the patient in a semi-sitting position during anesthesia induction and closely monitor for signs of airway obstruction.

61. SCENARIO: ANESTHETIC MANAGEMENT FOR INTRACRANIAL TUMOR RESECTION

A 45-year-old woman with a glioblastoma multiforme is scheduled for craniotomy. What special considerations should you have for anesthesia?

- **Answer**: Maintain stable hemodynamics, use brain-protective measures (e.g., mild hyperventilation to reduce intracranial pressure), and avoid hypotension.
- **Explanation**: Anesthesia for neurosurgery aims to maintain adequate cerebral perfusion pressure and minimize intracranial pressure.
- **Tip**: Use agents like propofol and remifentanil to allow for rapid emergence for neurological assessment postoperatively.

62. SCENARIO: PARANEOPLASTIC SYNDROME IN ANESTHESIA

A 55-year-old man with small cell lung cancer presents for resection. He has a history of muscle weakness and is diagnosed with Lambert-Eaton myasthenic syndrome. What are the anesthesia concerns?

- **Answer**: Avoid neuromuscular blockers if possible and titrate anesthetic agents carefully due to increased sensitivity.
- **Explanation**: Lambert-Eaton myasthenic syndrome results in sensitivity to neuromuscular blockers, with prolonged weakness after surgery.
- **Tip**: Consider using short-acting anesthetic agents and avoid long-acting muscle relaxants. Have a plan for post-operative ventilation if necessary.

63. SCENARIO: CHEMOTHERAPY-INDUCED CARDIOTOXICITY

A 50-year-old woman with a history of breast cancer treated with doxorubicin presents for mastectomy. She has developed heart failure. How would you manage her anesthesia?

- **Answer**: Use a balanced anesthesia technique, avoid myocardial depressants, and closely monitor hemodynamics with invasive monitoring.
- **Explanation**: Doxorubicin is associated with cardiomyopathy, and patients may have decreased cardiac reserve.
- **Tip**: Reduce fluid overload, avoid high-dose volatile agents, and consider the use of inotropes as needed.

64. SCENARIO: ANESTHETIC MANAGEMENT FOR A PATIENT WITH LEUKEMIA

A 12-year-old child with acute lymphoblastic leukemia (ALL) is undergoing surgery for central venous catheter insertion. What are the special considerations?

- **Answer**: Monitor for bleeding tendencies, avoid neuraxial anesthesia due to thrombocytopenia, and consider general anesthesia with careful airway management.
- **Explanation**: Leukemia can lead to pancytopenia, increasing the risk of bleeding, and infection.
- **Tip**: Ensure that platelet levels are adequate before surgery, and use blood products if necessary to reduce the risk of perioperative bleeding.

65. SCENARIO: RADIATION-INDUCED FIBROSIS IN AIRWAY MANAGEMENT

A 65-year-old man who underwent radiation therapy for laryngeal cancer presents for tracheostomy. His neck is stiff, and you anticipate a difficult airway. How would you manage it?

- **Answer**: Prepare for fiberoptic intubation or awake tracheostomy with local anesthesia due to expected airway fibrosis.
- **Explanation**: Radiation therapy can lead to airway fibrosis, making direct laryngoscopy difficult or impossible.
- **Tip**: Have a difficult airway cart ready, and consider the need for a surgical airway if endotracheal intubation fails.

66. SCENARIO: HYPERCALCEMIA IN A PATIENT WITH MULTIPLE MYELOMA

A 68-year-old man with multiple myeloma presents for vertebroplasty due to pathologic fractures. He has hypercalcemia with symptoms of lethargy and dehydration. How would you manage this?

- **Answer**: Correct dehydration with IV fluids, avoid volatile agents that may depress cardiac function, and monitor calcium levels during surgery.
- **Explanation**: Hypercalcemia can cause cardiac arrhythmias and hypotension, and patients often present dehydrated due to polyuria.
- **Tip**: Correct calcium levels preoperatively and monitor for signs of arrhythmias during anesthesia.

67. SCENARIO: PERIOPERATIVE MANAGEMENT IN A PATIENT WITH LUNG CANCER AND CHRONIC OBSTRUCTIVE PULMONARY DISEASE (COPD)

A 70-year-old smoker with lung cancer and severe COPD presents for lobectomy. What are the anesthesia concerns?

- **Answer**: Avoid high levels of oxygen, titrate ventilator settings to prevent hyperinflation, and monitor closely for respiratory depression post-operatively.
- **Explanation**: Patients with COPD are at high risk for perioperative respiratory complications, including hypercapnia and barotrauma.
- **Tip**: Use low tidal volumes, minimize volatile anesthetics, and provide adequate postoperative pain relief to prevent hypoventilation.

68. SCENARIO: INTRAOPERATIVE TUMOR LYSIS SYNDROME

A 58-year-old man with a large renal cell carcinoma develops sudden hyperkalemia, hypocalcemia, and arrhythmias during resection. What is your diagnosis and management?

- **Answer**: Suspect tumor lysis syndrome (TLS); treat with aggressive fluid resuscitation, manage hyperkalemia with calcium gluconate, and consider dialysis if necessary.
- **Explanation**: TLS occurs due to the rapid release of intracellular contents from tumor cells, leading to metabolic disturbances.
- **Tip**: Monitor electrolyte levels closely in patients with large tumor burdens, and ensure that supportive measures are available.

69. SCENARIO: HYPOTENSION IN A TRAUMA PATIENT WITH PELVIC FRACTURE

A 30-year-old male involved in a motor vehicle accident presents with a pelvic fracture and hypotension. How would you manage this trauma patient?

- **Answer**: Initiate fluid resuscitation with balanced crystalloids, apply a pelvic binder, and consider early blood transfusion if hypotension persists.

- **Explanation**: Pelvic fractures can lead to massive hemorrhage, and early stabilization of the pelvis is crucial to control bleeding.

- **Tip**: Avoid aggressive fluid resuscitation until surgical control of bleeding is achieved to prevent dilutional coagulopathy.

70. SCENARIO: AIRWAY MANAGEMENT IN A PATIENT WITH CERVICAL SPINE INJURY

A 45-year-old man involved in a diving accident presents with a suspected cervical spine injury. He requires intubation for airway protection. How would you approach airway management?

- **Answer**: Perform manual inline stabilization (MILS), avoid neck movement, and consider using a video laryngoscope or fiberoptic intubation.
- **Explanation**: Cervical spine injury requires careful airway management to avoid exacerbating spinal cord damage.
- **Tip**: Use a cervical collar and avoid chin lift or head tilt when securing the airway. Keep emergency tracheostomy equipment available.

71. SCENARIO: HEMORRHAGIC SHOCK FROM LIVER LACERATION

A 35-year-old woman involved in a high-speed motor vehicle accident presents with signs of hemorrhagic shock and a liver laceration. How would you manage fluid resuscitation?

- **Answer**: Initiate balanced crystalloid resuscitation, followed by early blood transfusion and damage control surgery.
- **Explanation**: Patients with liver lacerations are prone to significant bleeding, requiring rapid fluid and blood replacement to maintain hemodynamic stability.
- **Tip**: Use permissive hypotension until surgical control of bleeding is achieved to avoid exacerbating hemorrhage.

72. SCENARIO: MASSIVE TRANSFUSION PROTOCOL IN TRAUMA

A 28-year-old male with multiple stab wounds to the abdomen requires emergency laparotomy. He is receiving massive transfusion. What are your concerns?

- **Answer**: Monitor for coagulopathy, hypocalcemia, hyperkalemia, and hypothermia; administer blood products in a balanced ratio (e.g., 1:1:1 for RBCs, FFP, and platelets).
- **Explanation**: Massive transfusion can lead to dilutional coagulopathy, metabolic derangements, and hypothermia.
- **Tip**: Use warming devices, monitor electrolytes, and replace calcium as necessary to prevent complications.

73. SCENARIO: TENSION PNEUMOTHORAX DURING TRAUMA SURGERY

A 25-year-old male is undergoing exploratory laparotomy for abdominal trauma. He suddenly develops hypoxia, hypotension, and absent breath sounds on one side. What is your diagnosis and management?

- **Answer**: Suspect tension pneumothorax; immediately perform needle decompression followed by chest tube insertion.
- **Explanation**: Tension pneumothorax causes increased intrathoracic pressure, leading to decreased venous return and cardiovascular collapse.
- **Tip**: Have a high index of suspicion in trauma patients with sudden hemodynamic instability and provide rapid decompression to prevent cardiac arrest.

74. SCENARIO: ACUTE RESPIRATORY DISTRESS SYNDROME (ARDS)

A 52-year-old man is admitted to the ICU with pneumonia and develops ARDS. His oxygen saturation is 85% on 100% FiO2. What ventilation strategy would you use?

- **Answer**: Use low tidal volume ventilation (4-6 mL/kg ideal body weight), set PEEP (positive end-expiratory pressure) to maintain oxygenation, and limit plateau pressures to <30 cm H2O.
- **Explanation**: ARDS management requires lung-protective ventilation to avoid ventilator-induced lung injury (VILI) while optimizing oxygenation and ventilation.
- **Tip**: Monitor closely for hypercapnia and permissive hypoxia as trade-offs to avoid lung injury.

75. SCENARIO: WEANING FROM MECHANICAL VENTILATION

A 65-year-old female who was intubated for septic shock is now improving. You want to start weaning her off the ventilator. What is your approach?

- **Answer**: Conduct a spontaneous breathing trial (SBT) using pressure support ventilation or T-piece trial. Assess readiness for extubation based on mental status, airway protection, and respiratory parameters (e.g., rapid shallow breathing index, RSBI <105).

- **Explanation**: Weaning trials assess the patient's ability to breathe without full ventilator support, while balancing adequate oxygenation and ventilation.

- **Tip**: Extubation should be attempted only if the patient passes the SBT and has no other contraindications (e.g., strong cough, good mental status).

76. SCENARIO: VENTILATOR-ASSOCIATED PNEUMONIA (VAP)

A 70-year-old male intubated for respiratory failure develops fever, leukocytosis, and purulent secretions after 5 days on mechanical ventilation. What is your management?

- **Answer**: Suspect ventilator-associated pneumonia; obtain a respiratory culture, start empiric broad-spectrum antibiotics, and reassess once culture results are available.
- **Explanation**: VAP is a common ICU complication with increased morbidity and mortality. Early recognition and appropriate antibiotic therapy are key to management.
- **Tip**: Follow prevention strategies like elevation of the head of the bed, regular oral care, and minimizing sedation.

77. SCENARIO: PATIENT WITH CHRONIC OBSTRUCTIVE PULMONARY DISEASE (COPD) ON VENTILATOR

A 60-year-old male with COPD is intubated for acute respiratory failure. How would you set the ventilator?

- **Answer**: Use a low respiratory rate (10-12 breaths per minute), low tidal volume (6-8 mL/kg), and longer expiratory time to prevent air trapping (auto-PEEP).
- **Explanation**: COPD patients are prone to dynamic hyperinflation, leading to auto-PEEP and barotrauma. Setting appropriate ventilator parameters helps avoid these complications.
- **Tip**: Monitor closely for signs of auto-PEEP (e.g., rising plateau pressures) and adjust ventilator settings accordingly.

78. SCENARIO: PATIENT WITH ACUTE ASTHMA EXACERBATION ON MECHANICAL VENTILATION

A 28-year-old woman with severe asthma is intubated for status asthmaticus. How would you manage her on mechanical ventilation?

- **Answer**: Use low tidal volume (4-6 mL/kg), low respiratory rate (8-10 breaths/min), high inspiratory flow rates, and allow for prolonged expiration to prevent air trapping.
- **Explanation**: Asthma patients on mechanical ventilation are at high risk of dynamic hyperinflation, which can lead to barotrauma and hemodynamic compromise.
- **Tip**: Be cautious with sedation and paralytics as these patients often require higher doses to prevent asynchrony and control breathing patterns.

79. SCENARIO: VENTILATOR MANAGEMENT IN OBESE PATIENTS

A 45-year-old morbidly obese patient with a BMI of 42 is intubated following surgery. How would you set the ventilator for this patient?

- **Answer**: Use tidal volume based on ideal body weight (6-8 mL/kg), higher PEEP to maintain lung recruitment, and monitor closely for oxygenation and airway pressures.
- **Explanation**: Obese patients have reduced functional residual capacity and are at risk of atelectasis, necessitating adjustments in PEEP and tidal volumes.
- **Tip**: Be mindful of positional changes (e.g., head elevation) that may improve oxygenation and prevent lung collapse.

80. SCENARIO: PATIENT WITH SEPSIS ON MECHANICAL VENTILATION

A 55-year-old man with septic shock is on mechanical ventilation and requires high FiO2 to maintain oxygenation. His blood pressure remains low despite fluid resuscitation. What is your approach?

- **Answer**: Optimize oxygenation with lung-protective ventilation (low tidal volumes and appropriate PEEP), initiate vasopressor therapy (e.g., norepine) to maintain adequate perfusion, and ensure early, appropriate antibiotic therapy for sepsis management.
- **Explanation**: Sepsis induces a systemic inflammatory response, which can worsen ARDS and lead to refractory hypoxemia. Maintaining lung protection while supporting hemodynamics is critical.
- **Tip**: Titrate vasopressors to maintain MAP >65 mmHg, and ensure that fluid resuscitation is balanced to prevent fluid overload, especially in patients with ARDS.

81. SCENARIO: NON-INVASIVE VENTILATION (NIV) FOR ACUTE PULMONARY EDEMA

A 70-year-old female with heart failure presents with acute pulmonary edema, hypoxemia, and respiratory distress. She is placed on non-invasive ventilation (NIV). What settings would you use?

- **Answer**: Start with BiPAP (bilevel positive airway pressure) using inspiratory pressure (IPAP) of 10-12 cmH2O and expiratory pressure (EPAP/PEEP) of 5 cmH2O, titrate as needed to improve oxygenation and reduce work of breathing.
- **Explanation**: NIV provides positive pressure ventilation to improve alveolar recruitment, reduce pulmonary edema, and decrease the work of breathing.
- **Tip**: Monitor the patient for signs of improvement (e.g., reduced respiratory rate, improved oxygen saturation), and avoid NIV in patients with altered mental status or hemodynamic instability.

82. SCENARIO: VENTILATOR MANAGEMENT IN A PATIENT WITH TRAUMATIC BRAIN INJURY (TBI)

A 25-year-old male with a traumatic brain injury (TBI) is mechanically ventilated in the ICU. His intracranial pressure (ICP) is elevated. How would you adjust the ventilator?

- **Answer**: Use a low tidal volume (6-8 mL/kg), maintain normocapnia ($PaCO_2$ 35-40 mmHg), and avoid hyperventilation unless ICP is critically elevated.
- **Explanation**: Hyperventilation reduces CO_2, leading to vasoconstriction and lower ICP, but excessive reduction in $PaCO_2$ can cause cerebral ischemia.
- **Tip**: Optimize sedation, minimize PEEP to avoid raising ICP, and use invasive ICP monitoring to guide therapy.

83. SCENARIO: ACUTE HYPERCAPNIC RESPIRATORY FAILURE IN NEUROMUSCULAR DISEASE

A 35-year-old male with amyotrophic lateral sclerosis (ALS) presents with acute hypercapnic respiratory failure. He is intubated and placed on a ventilator. What settings should you consider?

- **Answer**: Use low tidal volume (6-8 mL/kg), high respiratory rate (12-16 breaths/min), and close monitoring of CO_2 levels to prevent hypercapnia. Consider non-invasive ventilation as a step-down strategy.
- **Explanation**: Neuromuscular patients are prone to hypoventilation and hypercapnia due to weakened respiratory muscles. Ventilation should be carefully adjusted to support gas exchange without overloading the respiratory muscles.
- **Tip**: Consider early tracheostomy in chronic neuromuscular conditions, and evaluate the need for long-term ventilator support.

84. SCENARIO: ACUTE POSTOPERATIVE PAIN MANAGEMENT

A 60-year-old woman undergoes an elective total knee arthroplasty. What multimodal analgesia strategy would you recommend for her postoperative pain management?

- **Answer**: Use a combination of opioids (e.g., hydromorphone), nonsteroidal anti-inflammatory drugs (NSAIDs) like ketorolac, and regional anesthesia such as a femoral nerve block.
- **Explanation**: Multimodal analgesia enhances pain control while minimizing opioid consumption, reducing the risk of side effects.
- **Tip**: Initiate the analgesic regimen preoperatively to optimize pain control in the immediate postoperative period.

85. SCENARIO: CHRONIC PAIN MANAGEMENT WITH NEUROPATHIC COMPONENT

A 45-year-old man presents with chronic pain due to diabetic neuropathy. What anesthetic techniques could be considered for managing his pain?

- **Answer**: Consider nerve blocks (e.g., lumbar plexus block), adjunctive medications (e.g., gabapentin), or implantable devices (e.g., spinal cord stimulation).
- **Explanation**: Neuropathic pain often requires a combination of pharmacological and interventional approaches for effective management.
- **Tip**: Assess the patient's overall pain profile and functional status to tailor the management plan.

86. SCENARIO: CANCER PAIN MANAGEMENT

A 70-year-old woman with metastatic breast cancer presents with uncontrolled pain despite high doses of oral opioids. How would you manage her pain more effectively?

- **Answer**: Consider starting a continuous intravenous (IV) opioid infusion, or switch to a transdermal fentanyl patch for better pain control.
- **Explanation**: Patients with cancer pain may require higher opioid dosages or alternative delivery methods to achieve adequate pain relief.
- **Tip**: Utilize the World Health Organization's pain ladder as a framework for escalating therapy and consider palliative care involvement for comprehensive management.

87. SCENARIO: LABOR ANALGESIA

A 28-year-old woman in labor requests pain relief. What anesthetic options are available, and what would you recommend?

- **Answer**: Recommend epidural analgesia for continuous pain relief, or consider intrathecal analgesia with opioids (e.g., fentanyl) for immediate pain control.
- **Explanation**: Epidural analgesia provides effective pain relief during labor while allowing the patient to remain mobile, depending on the local anesthetic used.
- **Tip**: Discuss the risks and benefits of each option, including potential side effects and the impact on labor progression.

88. SCENARIO: ACUTE PAIN MANAGEMENT IN A TRAUMA PATIENT

A 35-year-old male presents with severe pain from multiple rib fractures after a motorcycle accident. What analgesic techniques would you use?

- **Answer**: Initiate a multimodal approach including IV opioids, thoracic epidural analgesia, or intercostal nerve blocks for localized pain control.
- **Explanation**: Managing rib fracture pain is crucial to prevent respiratory complications, and regional techniques can effectively reduce opioid requirements.
- **Tip**: Monitor respiratory function closely, and consider supplemental oxygen therapy to ensure adequate ventilation.

89. SCENARIO: PAIN MANAGEMENT FOR A PATIENT WITH COMPLEX REGIONAL PAIN SYNDROME (CRPS)

A 50-year-old woman with CRPS in her right arm is experiencing severe, debilitating pain. What anesthetic interventions could be considered?

- **Answer**: Consider a sympathetic nerve block (e.g., stellate ganglion block) or spinal cord stimulation as part of the management plan.
- **Explanation**: CRPS often requires aggressive pain management strategies, including nerve blocks to interrupt pain pathways.
- **Tip**: Incorporate physical therapy and psychological support to address the multifaceted nature of CRPS.

90. SCENARIO: CHRONIC LOW BACK PAIN MANAGEMENT

A 40-year-old man with chronic low back pain due to degenerative disc disease seeks help. What anesthetic techniques could be employed?

- **Answer**: Consider epidural steroid injections, facet joint injections, or a trial of radiofrequency ablation for targeted pain relief.
- **Explanation**: Interventional pain management techniques can provide significant relief for chronic low back pain, especially when conservative measures fail.
- **Tip**: Regularly assess the effectiveness of interventions and modify the treatment plan based on the patient's response.

91. SCENARIO: PAIN CONTROL IN PATIENTS WITH SICKLE CELL CRISIS

A 30-year-old female with sickle cell disease presents in crisis with severe pain. What anesthetic management would you recommend?

- **Answer**: Administer IV opioids for rapid pain control, and consider adjunctive therapies such as ketorolac or gabapentin for better overall management.
- **Explanation**: Sickle cell crises are often accompanied by severe pain requiring prompt and aggressive analgesia.
- **Tip**: Monitor for potential complications, such as respiratory depression from high-dose opioids, and adjust treatment as necessary.

92. SCENARIO: REGIONAL ANESTHESIA FOR AMBULATORY SURGERY

A 50-year-old woman is scheduled for outpatient foot surgery. What regional anesthesia technique could be used for effective pain management postoperatively?

- **Answer**: Consider a popliteal nerve block for effective analgesia in the foot and ankle region.
- **Explanation**: Regional techniques like nerve blocks can provide excellent postoperative pain control and may facilitate faster recovery and discharge.
- **Tip**: Provide patients with clear postoperative instructions regarding block effects and when to seek help for any unusual symptoms.

93. SCENARIO: PEDIATRIC PAIN MANAGEMENT DURING SURGERY

A 10-year-old boy is undergoing a minor surgical procedure. What anesthetic approach would you recommend for his pain management?

- **Answer**: Use a combination of general anesthesia for the procedure and a regional block (e.g., a caudal block) for postoperative analgesia.
- **Explanation**: Combining general anesthesia with regional techniques enhances pain control while minimizing opioid use and associated side effects in children.
- **Tip**: Ensure that caregivers are educated about pain management and signs of inadequate analgesia postoperatively.

94. SCENARIO: PAIN MANAGEMENT IN PRETERM INFANT DURING PROCEDURES

A 28-week gestational age preterm infant is scheduled for a blood draw. What pain management strategies should be employed?

- **Answer**: Use a combination of non-pharmacological methods such as skin-to-skin contact (kangaroo care), sucrose solution, and provide gentle tactile stimulation.
- **Explanation**: Preterm infants are sensitive to pain, and using non-pharmacological methods can significantly reduce their distress during procedures.
- **Tip**: Administer sucrose just before the procedure, as it can provide analgesic effects when used in small doses.

95. SCENARIO: MANAGING PAIN IN A NEONATE WITH NEC

A 32-week gestational age infant diagnosed with necrotizing enterocolitis (NEC) is experiencing significant abdominal pain. What management options are appropriate?

- **Answer**: Administer opioids (e.g., morphine) for pain relief and provide supportive care, including careful monitoring of vital signs and bowel status.
- **Explanation**: Infants with NEC can experience severe pain; appropriate analgesia is crucial for comfort and can also support the healing process.
- **Tip**: Regularly assess pain levels using a validated neonatal pain scale (e.g., NIPS or PIPP).

96. SCENARIO: PAIN MANAGEMENT IN NEONATAL INTUBATION

A 1 kg infant is being intubated for respiratory distress. What analgesia should be considered?

- **Answer**: Provide intravenous (IV) fentanyl prior to intubation for rapid analgesia and sedation, along with a muscle relaxant if necessary.
- **Explanation**: Intubation can be distressing for neonates, and adequate analgesia and sedation are important to minimize pain and anxiety.
- **Tip**: Monitor the infant closely for respiratory depression following opioid administration.

97. SCENARIO: POSTOPERATIVE PAIN MANAGEMENT IN NEONATES

A neonate undergoes a surgical procedure for congenital diaphragmatic hernia repair. What pain management strategy should be employed postoperatively?

- **Answer**: Utilize continuous infusions of opioids (e.g., morphine) for pain control, along with regional anesthesia techniques such as a thoracic epidural if feasible.
- **Explanation**: Postoperative pain management is critical to promote recovery and minimize stress in neonates.
- **Tip**: Regularly assess the effectiveness of pain control and adjust medication dosages accordingly.

98. SCENARIO: PAIN MANAGEMENT FOR NEONATES WITH WITHDRAWAL SYMPTOMS

A neonate presents with signs of opioid withdrawal. What pain management approach should be used?

- **Answer**: Utilize a multidisciplinary approach including supportive care, oral morphine for withdrawal symptoms, and non-pharmacological interventions (e.g., swaddling, rocking).
- **Explanation**: Neonatal abstinence syndrome requires careful management to alleviate discomfort while monitoring for potential complications.
- **Tip**: Implement a scoring system to regularly assess the severity of withdrawal symptoms and guide treatment.

99. SCENARIO: MANAGING PAIN FROM PHOTOTHERAPY IN JAUNDICED NEONATES

A 2-day-old infant requires phototherapy for hyperbilirubinemia. What strategies can be employed to manage discomfort associated with phototherapy?

- **Answer**: Provide eye protection, ensure the infant is well-hydrated, and consider non-pharmacological interventions such as gentle rocking or soothing sounds.
- **Explanation**: While phototherapy is essential for treating jaundice, it can be uncomfortable; ensuring comfort is crucial.
- **Tip**: Use soft, dim lighting in the NICU to create a calming environment during phototherapy sessions.

100. SCENARIO: PAIN ASSESSMENT IN A CRITICALLY ILL NEONATE

A critically ill neonate is receiving invasive ventilation. How should pain be assessed and managed?

- **Answer**: Use a validated pain assessment tool for neonates (e.g., N-PASS or PIPP) and provide analgesics such as morphine based on pain assessment results.
- **Explanation**: Pain assessment in critically ill neonates can be challenging; using a structured tool ensures more accurate evaluation and appropriate management.
- **Tip**: Regularly re-evaluate pain levels, especially after changes in the clinical condition or following interventions.

101. SCENARIO: PAIN MANAGEMENT DURING CENTRAL LINE INSERTION

A preterm infant requires a central line for nutrition. What pain management strategies should be employed during the procedure?

- **Answer**: Administer local anesthetic (e.g., lidocaine) and provide sedation (e.g., midazolam) as appropriate, along with non-pharmacological techniques like swaddling.
- **Explanation**: Invasive procedures like central line insertion can cause significant pain; adequate analgesia is crucial for minimizing discomfort.
- **Tip**: Collaborate with the procedural team to ensure pain management strategies are in place before the procedure.

102. SCENARIO: MANAGING PAIN FOR A NEONATE WITH CARDIAC ISSUES

A neonate with congenital heart disease is experiencing pain post-cardiac surgery. What management plan should be implemented?

- **Answer**: Use a combination of opioids for analgesia (e.g., morphine) and consider regional anesthesia techniques if appropriate.
- **Explanation**: Cardiac surgery in neonates can be associated with significant pain; effective management is essential for recovery and stability.
- **Tip**: Monitor for signs of inadequate analgesia, such as increased heart rate or agitation, and adjust the pain management plan accordingly.

103. SCENARIO: LONG-TERM PAIN MANAGEMENT IN A NICU PATIENT

A 3-month-old infant with chronic lung disease in the NICU requires ongoing pain management. What approach should be taken?

- **Answer**: Implement a multimodal pain management strategy, including oral opioids for chronic pain and non-pharmacological measures (e.g., massage therapy).
- **Explanation**: Long-term pain management requires a comprehensive approach to improve quality of life while minimizing medication side effects.
- **Tip**: Involve a pain management specialist to create a tailored pain management plan considering the infant's evolving needs.

104. SCENARIO: ANESTHESIA FOR CORONARY ARTERY BYPASS GRAFTING (CABG)

A 65-year-old male is scheduled for CABG. He has a history of hypertension and diabetes. What anesthetic considerations should be taken into account?

- **Answer**: Use general anesthesia with a focus on maintaining hemodynamic stability. Consider using a beta-blocker preoperatively to manage heart rate and blood pressure.
- **Explanation**: Patients with cardiovascular comorbidities are at increased risk for intraoperative complications; maintaining hemodynamic parameters is crucial during surgery.
- **Tip**: Have a transesophageal echocardiogram (TEE) available for real-time assessment of cardiac function during the procedure.

105. SCENARIO: INTRAOPERATIVE HYPOTENSION DURING SURGERY

During aortic valve replacement surgery, the patient develops sudden hypotension. What could be the potential causes, and how would you manage it?

- **Answer**: Consider possible causes such as hypovolemia, cardiac dysfunction, or anesthetic agents. Administer intravenous fluids and vasopressors (e.g., norepinephrine) as needed.
- **Explanation**: Hypotension during cardiovascular surgery can arise from various factors; prompt identification and treatment are essential to prevent further complications.
- **Tip**: Continuously monitor blood pressure and cardiac output, and be prepared to adjust anesthesia and fluid management strategies.

106. SCENARIO: AWARENESS UNDER GENERAL ANESTHESIA

A 72-year-old patient undergoing aortic repair surgery reports vague memories of the surgical procedure postoperatively. What is your consideration regarding this phenomenon?

- **Answer**: This may indicate intraoperative awareness; review the anesthetic plan to ensure adequate depth of anesthesia (e.g., using BIS monitoring) during high-risk procedures.
- **Explanation**: Intraoperative awareness can occur, particularly in high-risk surgeries; preventive measures must be in place to avoid this distressing experience.
- **Tip**: Discuss the possibility of awareness with patients at higher risk and ensure they understand the monitoring used during surgery.

107. SCENARIO: MANAGEMENT OF ANTICOAGULATION IN CARDIAC SURGERY

A patient on warfarin presents for elective mitral valve surgery. What preoperative management should be done regarding anticoagulation?

- **Answer**: Hold warfarin several days prior to surgery, and bridge with low molecular weight heparin (LMWH) if indicated, monitoring INR closely.
- **Explanation**: Proper management of anticoagulation is critical to minimize the risk of bleeding during surgery while preventing thromboembolic events.
- **Tip**: Communicate with the surgical team about the anticoagulation plan and confirm that the INR is within target range prior to the procedure.

108. SCENARIO: CARDIOPULMONARY BYPASS COMPLICATIONS

During a surgery requiring cardiopulmonary bypass (CPB), the patient experiences hemodynamic instability. What complications should be considered?

- **Answer**: Potential complications include hypothermia, hemodilution, electrolyte imbalances, and pump-related issues. Rapidly assess the patient's hemodynamic status and adjust CPB settings as needed.
- **Explanation**: CPB can lead to a variety of physiological changes; maintaining stable hemodynamics during this period is vital.
- **Tip**: Regularly monitor and manage temperature, blood pressure, and blood gas levels during CPB to minimize complications.

109. SCENARIO: ACUTE CORONARY SYNDROME (ACS) DURING SURGERY

A patient undergoing cardiac surgery develops signs of acute coronary syndrome (ACS). What management steps should be taken?

- **Answer**: Evaluate the patient's hemodynamics and consider administering nitroglycerin for chest pain, along with additional anti-anginal medications as needed. Maintain hemodynamic stability and prepare for potential revascularization.
- **Explanation**: ACS during surgery can complicate the procedure; prompt identification and management are critical to optimize outcomes.
- **Tip**: Collaborate closely with the surgical team and cardiology to ensure a coordinated response to manage ACS effectively.

110. SCENARIO: HEMOLYTIC REACTION DURING CARDIAC SURGERY

During surgery, a patient experiences a hemolytic transfusion reaction. What immediate actions should be taken?

- **Answer**: Stop the transfusion immediately, maintain venous access with normal saline, notify the surgical team, and treat symptoms (e.g., fever, hypotension) as necessary. Send blood samples for further analysis.
- **Explanation**: Hemolytic reactions can lead to significant morbidity; rapid recognition and management are crucial to prevent complications.
- **Tip**: Review transfusion protocols and ensure all staff are trained to recognize and respond to transfusion reactions.

111. SCENARIO: INTRAOPERATIVE CARDIAC ARREST

A patient undergoing valve replacement surgery experiences cardiac arrest. What is the immediate management protocol?

- **Answer**: Initiate CPR immediately, call for help, and prepare for defibrillation if indicated. Administer epinephrine and consider advanced airway management as needed.
- **Explanation**: Intraoperative cardiac arrest requires prompt and coordinated efforts to restore circulation and airway management.
- **Tip**: Conduct regular simulations and drills for the surgical and anesthesia teams to ensure readiness for emergencies like cardiac arrest.

112. SCENARIO: ANESTHESIA FOR CRANIOTOMY

A 55-year-old female is scheduled for a craniotomy to remove a brain tumor. What anesthetic considerations should be taken into account?

- **Answer**: Use general anesthesia with a focus on brain protection, maintaining normal hemodynamics, and adequate intracranial pressure (ICP) monitoring.
- **Explanation**: Neurological surgeries require careful management of anesthesia to prevent fluctuations in blood pressure and ICP, which can affect surgical outcomes.
- **Tip**: Consider using dexmedetomidine for sedation, as it provides analgesia and has minimal respiratory depression.

113. SCENARIO: INTRAOPERATIVE NEUROMONITORING

During a spinal surgery, intraoperative neuromonitoring indicates changes in motor evoked potentials. What actions should the anesthesiologist take?

- **Answer**: Notify the surgical team immediately, assess blood pressure and anesthetic depth, and consider reducing or modifying the anesthetic agents to optimize neuromonitoring.
- **Explanation**: Changes in motor evoked potentials can indicate potential injury to the spinal cord or nerve roots, necessitating immediate intervention.
- **Tip**: Have a protocol in place for rapid response to changes in neuromonitoring during surgeries.

114. SCENARIO: POSTOPERATIVE CEREBRAL EDEMA

A patient undergoes a craniectomy and develops signs of cerebral edema in the postoperative period. What management strategies should be employed?

- **Answer**: Administer corticosteroids (e.g., dexamethasone) to reduce inflammation and edema, and consider hyperosmolar therapy (e.g., mannitol) if indicated.
- **Explanation**: Cerebral edema can lead to increased ICP, necessitating prompt management to prevent neurological complications.
- **Tip**: Monitor neurological status closely and consider imaging studies to assess for complications like hematoma formation.

115. SCENARIO: SEIZURE MANAGEMENT IN NEUROSURGERY

A patient with a history of seizures is undergoing a temporal lobectomy. How should the anesthetic plan be adjusted?

- **Answer**: Use an appropriate anticonvulsant (e.g., levetiracetam) preoperatively, maintain stable anesthesia, and ensure rapid recovery to prevent seizures postoperatively.

- **Explanation**: Patients with a history of seizures may require additional measures to prevent perioperative seizure activity, which can complicate recovery.

- **Tip**: Have seizure medications readily available and establish a clear postoperative seizure management plan.

116. SCENARIO: ANESTHESIA FOR SPINAL FUSION

A 30-year-old male is undergoing spinal fusion for severe back pain. What regional anesthesia technique could be utilized?

- **Answer**: Consider a combined spinal-epidural technique for intraoperative analgesia and postoperative pain management.
- **Explanation**: The combined technique provides effective analgesia and may allow for faster recovery with reduced opioid consumption.
- **Tip**: Ensure that the patient is monitored closely for any signs of complications related to regional anesthesia, such as hematoma or infection.

117. SCENARIO: ANESTHESIA FOR THYROIDECTOMY

A 45-year-old woman is scheduled for a total thyroidectomy. What are the anesthetic considerations for this procedure?

- **Answer**: Use general anesthesia with careful airway management, and ensure availability of equipment for potential airway complications due to swelling or hematoma.
- **Explanation**: Thyroid surgeries can lead to airway difficulties due to edema or hematoma formation; preparedness is key to managing these risks.
- **Tip**: Position the patient in a way that facilitates airway access, and consider using a neuromuscular blocking agent for optimal intubation conditions.

118. SCENARIO: HYPERPARATHYROIDISM SURGERY COMPLICATIONS

A patient undergoing parathyroidectomy for hyperparathyroidism develops hypotension during the procedure. What could be the underlying causes?

- **Answer**: Possible causes include hypovolemia, sympathetic blockade from anesthesia, or vasodilation due to anesthetic agents. Administer IV fluids and vasopressors if necessary.
- **Explanation**: Understanding the cause of hypotension is crucial for timely and appropriate management to maintain hemodynamic stability during surgery.
- **Tip**: Continuously monitor blood pressure and fluid status, especially in patients with electrolyte imbalances due to hyperparathyroidism.

119. SCENARIO: POSTOPERATIVE HYPOPARATHYROIDISM

After a total thyroidectomy, a patient exhibits symptoms of hypoparathyroidism. What management strategies should be implemented?

- **Answer**: Monitor serum calcium levels and administer calcium supplementation and vitamin D as needed to manage symptoms of hypocalcemia.
- **Explanation**: Damage to parathyroid glands during thyroid surgery can lead to hypoparathyroidism, requiring careful monitoring and management of calcium levels.
- **Tip**: Educate the patient about signs of hypocalcemia and the need for follow-up to monitor calcium levels postoperatively.

120. SCENARIO: CARDIOVASCULAR INSTABILITY DURING ENDOCRINE SURGERY

A patient with a history of adrenal insufficiency undergoes adrenalectomy and develops cardiovascular instability. What management steps should be taken?

- **Answer**: Administer IV fluids and consider hydrocortisone for adrenal support. Monitor blood pressure and heart rate closely and be prepared to initiate vasopressor therapy if necessary.
- **Explanation**: Patients with adrenal insufficiency are at risk for adrenal crisis during surgery; proactive management is essential.
- **Tip**: Ensure that the surgical team is aware of the patient's history and that protocols for managing adrenal insufficiency are in place.

121. SCENARIO: ANESTHESIA FOR PATIENT WITH CHRONIC KIDNEY DISEASE (CKD)

A 70-year-old patient with stage 3 CKD is scheduled for elective hip surgery. What anesthetic considerations should be made?

- **Answer**: Use general anesthesia with careful attention to fluid management and avoidance of nephrotoxic agents. Monitor renal function closely during the perioperative period.

- **Explanation**: Patients with CKD have altered pharmacokinetics for many drugs, making them more susceptible to the effects of anesthetics and potential nephrotoxicity.

- **Tip**: Avoid NSAIDs and certain antibiotics that may exacerbate renal impairment; consider using regional anesthesia if appropriate.

122. SCENARIO: INTRAOPERATIVE HEMOLYSIS IN A DIALYSIS PATIENT

During surgery, a patient with end-stage renal disease (ESRD) develops signs of hemolysis after receiving a blood transfusion. What should the anesthesiologist do?

- **Answer**: Stop the transfusion immediately, maintain venous access with normal saline, and notify the surgical team. Perform a workup to assess for hemolytic reaction.
- **Explanation**: Hemolytic reactions can lead to serious complications, especially in patients with renal disorders, and require rapid intervention to prevent further harm.
- **Tip**: Ensure that blood products are properly matched and screened prior to administration, especially in patients with a history of transfusion reactions.

123. SCENARIO: POSTOPERATIVE MANAGEMENT OF A PATIENT WITH ACUTE KIDNEY INJURY (AKI)

A patient presents with AKI following major abdominal surgery. What management strategies should be implemented?

- **Answer**: Monitor renal function (creatinine and electrolytes), ensure adequate hydration, and avoid nephrotoxic medications. Consider diuretics if fluid overload occurs.

- **Explanation**: Early identification and management of AKI are crucial to minimize long-term renal damage and complications.

- **Tip**: Consult nephrology for guidance on management strategies, especially if there is no improvement in renal function.

124. SCENARIO: ANESTHESIA FOR RENAL TRANSPLANTATION

A patient is undergoing renal transplantation. What anesthetic considerations should be addressed for optimal outcomes?

- **Answer**: Use general anesthesia with careful monitoring of hemodynamics and fluid balance. Prepare for rapid changes in blood volume and electrolyte levels during and after surgery.

- **Explanation**: Renal transplantation can cause significant hemodynamic shifts and fluid changes; careful management is critical to prevent complications.

- **Tip**: Have renal replacement therapy (e.g., dialysis) available postoperatively in case of acute graft dysfunction.

125. SCENARIO: MANAGING ELECTROLYTE IMBALANCE IN A DIALYSIS PATIENT

A dialysis patient undergoing elective surgery presents with elevated potassium levels (hyperkalemia). What should be the immediate management?

- **Answer**: Administer calcium gluconate or calcium chloride to stabilize the myocardium, followed by insulin and glucose to shift potassium into cells. Consider hemodialysis if potassium levels remain high.
- **Explanation**: Hyperkalemia poses a significant risk during surgery due to its potential to cause cardiac arrhythmias; prompt management is essential.
- **Tip**: Ensure continuous cardiac monitoring during the perioperative period for patients with known electrolyte imbalances.

126. SCENARIO: ANESTHESIA FOR LIVER TRANSPLANTATION

A 60-year-old male with end-stage liver disease is scheduled for a liver transplant. What specific anesthetic considerations should be taken into account?

- **Answer**: Use general anesthesia with careful monitoring of coagulation status and fluid management. Consider preoperative optimization of liver function and addressing potential portal hypertension.
- **Explanation**: Patients with liver disease are at risk for coagulopathy and hemodynamic instability; thus, managing fluid balance and bleeding risk is critical.
- **Tip**: Have blood products readily available and be prepared for rapid transfusions during surgery.

127. SCENARIO: POSTOPERATIVE COMPLICATIONS FOLLOWING KIDNEY TRANSPLANT

A patient develops acute rejection of a transplanted kidney 48 hours postoperatively. What immediate management steps should be taken?

- **Answer**: Administer high-dose corticosteroids (e.g., methylprednisolone) to manage acute rejection and ensure close monitoring of renal function and electrolytes.
- **Explanation**: Acute rejection requires prompt treatment to preserve graft function; corticosteroids are the first-line therapy for this condition.
- **Tip**: Collaborate with the transplant nephrologist to determine the most appropriate immunosuppressive therapy postoperatively.

128. SCENARIO: INTRAOPERATIVE ANAPHYLAXIS DURING HEART TRANSPLANT

During a heart transplant, the patient experiences signs of anaphylaxis after receiving a blood transfusion. What should be the immediate course of action?

- **Answer**: Stop the transfusion immediately, provide high-flow oxygen, administer epinephrine, and prepare for airway management if needed.
- **Explanation**: Anaphylaxis is a critical emergency that requires rapid response to prevent cardiovascular collapse, especially in a vulnerable transplant patient.
- **Tip**: Ensure that all team members are aware of the signs of anaphylaxis and are trained in emergency response protocols.

129. SCENARIO: MANAGEMENT OF HYPERGLYCEMIA IN A PANCREAS TRANSPLANT

A patient undergoing simultaneous pancreas and kidney transplantation develops hyperglycemia during the procedure. What management strategies should be employed?

- **Answer**: Administer intravenous insulin to manage blood glucose levels and monitor for hypoglycemia postoperatively as the pancreas begins to function.
- **Explanation**: Hyperglycemia can occur due to stress response and medications; tight glycemic control is essential in transplant patients to promote graft function.
- **Tip**: Continue to monitor blood glucose levels closely during recovery, and adjust insulin therapy as needed based on the patient's response.

130. SCENARIO: POSTOPERATIVE CARE FOR LUNG TRANSPLANT PATIENT

A lung transplant recipient develops acute respiratory distress postoperatively. What are the potential causes and management strategies?

- **Answer**: Possible causes include primary graft dysfunction, pneumonia, or fluid overload. Management should involve optimizing ventilation and oxygenation, and considering diuretics if fluid overload is suspected.
- **Explanation**: Postoperative respiratory complications are common in lung transplant patients; prompt recognition and intervention are crucial for recovery.
- **Tip**: Implement a protocol for routine assessment of respiratory function and signs of rejection or infection in the immediate postoperative period.

ABOUT THE AUTHOR

Essam Abdelhakim

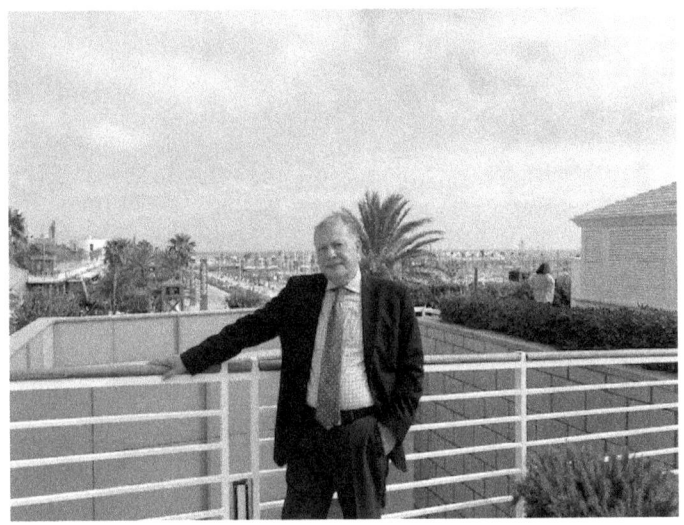

Senior Consultant and expert in Medical Education

www.ingramcontent.com/pod-product-compliance
Lightning Source LLC
Chambersburg PA
CBHW050257230526
45471CB00005B/1920